WHEN I'M NOT
ME ANYMORE

WHEN I'M NOT ME ANYMORE

A Pre-Dementia Love Letter to My Daughters

RHONDA HOFFMAN

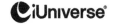

WHEN I'M NOT ME ANYMORE
A Pre-Dementia Love Letter to My Daughters

iUniverse books may be ordered through booksellers or by contacting:

iUniverse
1663 Liberty Drive
Bloomington, IN 47403
www.iuniverse.com
1-800-Authors (1-800-288-4677)

Because of the dynamic nature of the Internet, any web addresses or links contained in this book may have changed since publication and may no longer be valid. The views expressed in this work are solely those of the author and do not necessarily reflect the views of the publisher, and the publisher hereby disclaims any responsibility for them.

Any people depicted in stock imagery provided by Getty Images are models, and such images are being used for illustrative purposes only. Certain stock imagery © Getty Images.

ISBN: 978-1-5320-8035-7 (sc)
ISBN: 978-1-5320-8036-4 (e)

Library of Congress Control Number: 2019914806

Print information available on the last page.

iUniverse rev. date: 11/07/2019

This book is lovingly dedicated to my daughters, Rebecca and Rachel, in memory of my mother, Eileen. If her struggles become mine, I trust that you will find guidance in these pages and the assurance that, if the day comes that, I don't know your faces, I will always know your hearts.

CONTENTS

PREFACE

My mom took her last breath at ninety-three years of age. Unfortunately, the real Eileen left us years before in the form of a lost train of thought here or a forgotten word there. We thought it was a natural by-product of ageing but, in retrospect, it was dementia taking hold.

Near the end, when she lost interest in most of the world around her, it was hard remembering that she wasn't always like that. She was once a toddler learning to walk; a vibrant young woman falling in love; and a strong, quiet force alongside my father in their sixty years of ministry. But when our conversations became shallow and bizarre and lacked connection, the painful realization that something had changed took hold. I wondered if there was anything she would have wanted to say to me, knowing that our time left together would be so short. Perhaps there was a secret she once thought she couldn't tell, but I never found out because her jumbled thoughts were a mixture of facts and fiction by then.

It was a privilege for my sisters and me as we helped Dad keep Mom at home and care for her. Being a family means living each day without keeping score of who did what for whom; but that last stage of mom's life allowed us to give back to her, in a tangible way, the love and care that she gave us over a lifetime. Our lack of understanding about dementia meant we had to learn as we went along, and sometimes going through the same scenario again and again was the only way to discover the best course of action. This created frustration and aggravation before the reality and sadness of what was happening sunk in. The game for Mom had changed, and we girls were still using the old rules to make sense of things—which didn't get us very far.

I don't claim to be any kind of expert on dementia or Alzheimer's disease, but I have seen firsthand the effects they had on my mom and our family. My goal for this book is to share thoughts from my heart to kindred spirits on a similar journey and to prepare my daughters for what may come.

The fact that Mom had dementia doesn't mean I will get it, but I've often thought about what my daughters may have to deal with if I go down the same path. What would I want them to know? If I could have another lucid conversation with my mom, what might she want to tell me, and what would I want to hear from her?

With this in mind, this book is first and foremost for my daughters. Like many parents, I often wished children came with instruction manuals, but I also felt the same way when adjusting to the changes in Mom. I hope that down the road my girls will recognize the behaviors mentioned here and use that understanding to help them cope. This collection of thoughts and instruction is a love letter to my daughters to express myself completely so that, if the day comes when words elude me, they will find my heart in these pages.

Even though everyone's journey is different, there is much about dementia that can be predicted and mitigated. With the staggering increase of dementia and Alzheimer's disease among baby boomers, I realized that I am not alone in this journey and that my experience could perhaps help others. For this reason, I am sharing these very personal musings with you in addition to my daughters. We will talk about the initial frustration of our loved one forgetting something we just told them or stopping mid-story to say, "Now why was I telling you that?" Time loses meaning when our loved one has nowhere to go and all day to get there, forgetting that we still have commitments, appointments, and things to do. We experience a sense of time travel when *where* we are becomes *when* we are as their memories from the past get jumbled up in their happenings of today. We will look at how their language changes bringing about surprising and sometimes disturbing conversations as the filters from the past wane and we see them in their uncut glory.

Until there is a cure for dementia or Alzheimer's disease, there are ways to soften their effects on us; that's why you will find some tips and encouragement here as well. In the appendix, I offer journaling questions to encourage parents and their children to capture thoughts and stories before they are lost forever. My hope is that we can be remembered, even when we ourselves forget.

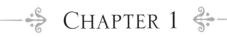

CHAPTER 1

A LOVE LETTER

Dearest Rebecca and Rachel,

I am writing this while I am still in full command of my faculties; I hope that as I age, my mental capacities will remain undiminished. In the later years of Grandma's life, we all came to a new understanding of how dementia affects not only those afflicted with it but everyone around them as well. I am doing what I can now to stave off the onset of dementia, but I know that very little in life works out the way we plan, so I am giving this book to you as a gift in case the time comes when my mind fails me. If or when this happens, I need you to know that I'm not "me" anymore.

I will have forgotten what it means to be me, and I will have a diminished understanding of the world and my place in it. When I tell you that everything is changing, I mean everything is changing for all of us. This is not a solitary condition, as it affects everything from how we communicate to how we spend our time: we will experience loss on a whole new level. I will become a familiar stranger who looks like your mom but behaves and speaks like someone else.

I know it's probably hard to believe, looking at me now, but I was full of dreams, knew love and passion, and enjoyed being a woman. I was no different from you, so when time runs its course and I am no longer vital, be patient with me. I never dreamed that I would sit with you and have nothing to say, but that will become a common occurrence. My mental processes will no longer be sharp, and when you feel frustrated because I've just asked you the same question three times, please remember that I am trying to connect. I may not be successful, but I am trying. Down the road, if I share words of anger or frustration with you, they are coming from someone I don't recognize. If I lash out, it will be because I am afraid or feeling vulnerable. It isn't easy going from independence and strength to dependency and frailty, but always remember that the last thing I ever want to do is hurt you.

In times when I may not remember your face, know that I still hold you in my heart. I gave you life, and you gave it back to me with every hug, every movie afternoon, and every moment of laughter.

I pray if I lose my memories that the bad ones go first—like the heartbreaks of realizing that life didn't turn out the way it was supposed to, and dreams that never took flight; like the trespasses of those who hurt us, intentionally or not, and betrayals of those we entrusted our hearts to who weren't worthy of that trust. Those heartbreaks just aren't worth holding on to because they rob us of time that could go toward enjoying life and building good memories. Remember this for yourself, even if I don't.

I believe you know that I did my very best for you with the knowledge and resources I had at the time. I walked my talk and tried to be a good example for you. I taught you God's ways and, once you were an adult, I did my best to let you make your own choices and live with the rewards and consequences that came with them. So many times I wanted to try to keep you from choosing poorly, but I bit my tongue… most of the time. It made me feel so good when you asked for my help with something. We never outgrow the need to be needed. Remember that, even now with those around you.

One thing I hope I never, ever forget is how much we laughed together. We enjoyed each other's company, which is more than a lot of mothers and daughters can say. I am so blessed to have shared years of love and laughter with you both. What great times we had snuggled up in my bed when you were young, making up stories, and laughing until we cried. So many of those jokes lasted all through your adult years and make us smile even now. Part of the deterioration of my communication skills is that I won't understand humor the way I used to, and this will be a great loss for all of us. If this occurs, think back on the years and years of fun we had and remember them for me.

You are my world, but don't make me yours. Let me be part of your life but don't let my needs consume you. Being a caregiver is the hardest job, and I never want you to resent being in that position. Know there is no guilt in letting someone else help me with daily living. There are many people out there who can take care of me, but only you can be my daughters and friends. This is the way I want it to be.

Speaking of these matters in a future tense makes it too easy to fall back on the idea that these challenges only happen to other people and that we, therefore, won't have to worry about them. With this in mind, this book is written in the present tense from an imagined time when I have already begun the descent into the land of forgetfulness. The chapters are short, but I trust that they will help you gain insight into the strange world of dementia that we may find ourselves navigating.

Lastly, we hear stories of people regretting that the last words they said to a loved one were of anger or disinterest, not knowing they would never see that person again. If that is ever the case with us, please let go of that regret. I know you love me, and a few harsh words would never cancel out the lifetime of love you have given me. Even if I'm not me anymore, the part that sometimes remembers will feel your love and laughter and warmth and kindness still. Few people have known love the way you have loved me, and I will carry that with me always.

Love always,

Mom

CHAPTER 2

"OF ALL THE THINGS I'VE LOST, I MISS MY MIND THE MOST"

When you are with me, and see me forgetful and confused, I want you to think about what dementia is like. A metaphor, given to me by the Alzheimer's Society of Alberta, is one of a truck driving along its route with a full load of memories. As it comes around a corner, a box falls off and lies in the middle of the road, which means a car behind the truck—a thought in this case—must swerve to miss it. That was what was happening in the beginning when I struggled for a word or lost my train of thought. As that truck continued on the route, it kept dropping more boxes, making the roadway between my thoughts more and more congested. Pretty soon it was a complete obstacle course, and I was unable to find my way because, with my life scattered across the road, I couldn't locate the box that held any particular memory. That included my memories about how to think logically, about how to brush my teeth, or that I needed to brush them at all.

I recognize that this now poses challenges and more than a few uncomfortable situations for you; but in all of what is happening, remember that it affects me too. It's frustrating to know that I know something but can't think of what it is. It will be a relief for me if the day comes when I don't know that I should know something. This won't ease your frustration because you will still have the capacity to recall what you need to, and my inability might not make sense to you.

> Things that seem so simple to you and were so simple for me at one time are now foreign to me. If you can keep that in mind, it might help you more easily navigate our time together.

I don't know why some people struggle with losing their mental faculties and some don't, but I do know it is no one's fault. Yes, many things can be done to mitigate this condition, and I believe I did my best in that regard; but whatever brought me here, here is where I am. I understand that it can be frustrating for you, but don't be angry. It won't change anything and will only rob you of time and energy. Let's spend today the best we can, even if I won't remember it tomorrow.

When you look into these eyes, the ones that seem to look through you now rather than at you, remember that they once sparkled with life. They softened at the sight of your beautiful face. They shone with pride when you got on the bus for your first day of kindergarten, at your first recital, and on the day you graduated. These eyes have seen so much life, both good and bad, and those moments are snapshots that replay in my memory. If enough of my faculties remain to notice these memories leave me, it means I am feeling that loss every day now. Imagine knowing your life is slipping away one piece at a time and that nothing you do can retrieve it. These eyes that have cried a million tears of both heartbreak and joy are now looking out but seeing nothing. If you look closely enough, you will still see me in the far recesses. There, in my own private world, I am reliving our life together and all of the wonder God let me see through you. When you are feeling sad because we've been robbed of what we had, read through these pages and remember for both of us. I loved you before you were born, and I will love you into life beyond.

CHAPTER 3

MY TRAIN (OF THOUGHT) HAS LEFT THE STATION

I did my best in the years leading up to this time to make this season of my life one of peace and contentment. Hopefully, the regrets of the past will not consume me, making me angry and miserable. No one grows up thinking they are going to be that crabby old lady—including that crabby old lady.

My ability to understand and process information is greatly impaired, and I now need instructions for the simple tasks that I used to do without even knowing it. Putting on my blouse has become a ten-step ordeal with me having to process—*really* process—every step. My struggle with this is going to seem ridiculous to you, but it is very real to me, and it becomes more of a burden for me each passing day. Multitasking is a thing of the past, as every action and thought requires total concentration, and this is if I don't forget what I am doing in the first place.

My decreasing ability to process my thoughts can lead to many misunderstandings and become a source of mutual frustration. If I am having a hard time finding a word, don't be too quick to fill it in for me. I took pride in being independent, and if a thought hangs in mid-sentence, let us not be concerned with it because it doesn't matter anymore. Unfortunately, this condition will only get worse; there is no coming back from dementia yet.

Our communication is getting more difficult partly because I am hard of hearing, but, even more, because I am not able to process…your…words…as…quickly…as… I… used…to. The way you speak to me makes a big difference in that keeping your phrases simple and loud and saying them slowly sets me up to win at giving you a correct answer. Try to keep your sentences short and try not to mind repeating yourself several times if that is what it takes. By the time you have finished saying a fifteen-word sentence to me, I'll still be working on the fourth word, so it is very important for you to slow down your speech. Again, I know how frustrating this will be until you master it, and I know you will feel silly speaking this way, but it will make a world of difference for us. If I only hear part of what you say, I will make up the rest. Chances are very good that it will not match what you said, and you can see where this will lead to some very interesting outcomes. It takes a lot for me to follow a conversation now; so if I have trouble staying on topic or interject with a *non sequitur*, don't wonder where it came from. It made sense according to what I thought I heard.

There are other ways to ease our communication together. Limiting distractions, like the radio or television in the background, can help a great deal. The same goes for closing the windows if noise is coming in. My mind can only tolerate so much at a time now, and the noises all blur together; making it impossible for me to separate them and make sense of what you are saying.

Even though we may have discussed something, it doesn't mean I will remember it later, so leaving notes for me as visual reminders can greatly help me function.

Feel free to use hand gestures and body language while we are talking to make your point. The movement helps me engage more and possibly interpret something I didn't quite hear. As my speech becomes less clear, you may have difficulty understanding what I am trying to say. If this happens, draw upon my past experiences and what you know about me to help us both make sense of the message I am trying to get across. Dementia Charades will become our new game.

At some point, communication between us may no longer be verbal at all. This doesn't mean I don't want to hear your sweet voice, but rather that most of our interactions will be physical. At any age, a tender touch says much more than words can convey, so holding my hand or stroking the inside of my arm will let me know that you are there and that I am still loved. At this stage, what you'll be saying won't mean as much as how you are saying it. The tone and rhythm of your voice will let your affection shine through and help me to feel safe and relaxed.

It may be hard to reconcile that silence is not a divide between us. It probably drives you nuts that I can just sit and stare into space, looking at nothing in particular with no need for outside stimulation. My sense of adventure is long gone, and I have no desire to do anything, which is another reminder of how much I have changed. Nonetheless, it is where I am, and it will be new to me too.

When you try to get me involved in hobbies or visiting friends, I am not the least bit interested. It's not because I'm stubborn; these activities simply don't mean what they used to for me. Period. I am probably bowing out of social situations also because it's harder or impossible for me to follow the conversations or humor of those around me, making me feel less and less like I fit in. Add in my hearing loss and the fact that it takes me longer to process the banter at the table, and it should make sense why I choose to withdraw. This is a lonely and frustrating place for me.

Imagine being at our Christmas dinner table with the whole family gathered around, but you are sitting inside a plastic bubble. You can see everyone talking and laughing but can't make out what is so funny. You can see that they are addressing you at times but they-are-speaking-so-fast-that-you-are-unable-to-process-what-they-are-saying. You're part of the group but not part of it at the same time, which makes it easier to sit with your head down and focus on your meal than to try to engage. Now you have a good idea of how I feel.

I am not interested in movie afternoons anymore, mostly because I'm not able to follow the plots and everyone talks too quickly; but putting on a relaxing DVD with scenes and sounds of nature may be soothing for me. Playing calm music with the sound of rain is something I would enjoy. Borrowing from poet William Congreve, music soothes the savage (and demented) breast. This isn't to say we are confined to staying indoors and, though it's harder for me to get around, hopefully I still like going for walks, and that could be therapeutic for both of us.

You know how much I loved reading, and I sure hope that all those self-help books came through and I am now a wealthy, svelte, multilingual, award-winning, bestselling author and business mogul. If not, I will have to file that under the heading of "it's not the destination, but the journey." Reading may have gone the way of the dodo for me and, if so, the death of this favorite pastime of mine could be two-fold. As mentioned before, I am not able to follow the plots anymore and my age may also be showing up in the form of double vision. This is common in seniors and can often be corrected with special glasses through a trip to an ophthalmologist. Still, you can feel free to leave a sappy romance novel by my bedside. I wouldn't want to waste a lucid moment should one arise.

CHAPTER 4

NOWHERE TO GO AND ALL DAY TO GET THERE

As the productive members of society I raised you to be, I know your lives are full of people you love and ever-present commitments. Please don't be impatient with me when I am moving slowly. Part of it is physical—my body can no longer cash the cheques my mind is still writing—but the other part is that I have nowhere else I need to be. All of those appointments, lunches, and duties that once made up my life have fallen by the wayside. Things like that don't even enter my mind anymore.

For so many years, I rushed from one place to the next, trying to fit everything in. But somewhere along the way, I can't even tell you when it was, I had nowhere to go. You were self-sufficient and didn't need me like you used to. It's a strange thing to no longer be needed. Even with all my other responsibilities, I lived for you. Because I did my job well, you started living your own life. My work was done, and it was time to move on to something else.

We work so long and hard while we look forward to our Golden Years, when we get to put aside our work-life and slip into retirement; but when it is upon us, it can be frightening. It feels odd not having deadlines and commitments. I'm often in limbo, not sure of what I should be doing. With my working life done, there was no need to get up in the mornings anymore; but I was never able to convince my body and reset my internal clock. I have all the time in the world now, but little control over how to use it.

> I can no longer choose where to go and how to get there. Stop for a moment to imagine that. It is hard to accept that someone else should dictate your movements. Being told where to go and when is humiliating for someone who used to be so independent. Once the driver, I am now relegated to being a passenger, with little or no say in what happens to me. I'm frustrated and feel small, and there's a good chance I can't even express those feelings effectively now.

My advice to you is to get involved, make friends, join clubs, volunteer. Although this is harder to do as you get older, it's never too late to start. When the time comes to pack away your tools and relax, don't underestimate how important having somewhere else to go will be. It is important to enjoy your own company, but it will be essential for you to have friends to enjoy when this time comes.

I understand that just because my life has slowed down, it doesn't mean yours has or will need to. For now, I will try to remember that you still have things to do, places to go, and people to see. I'll simply be glad that I am one of those people. It won't make me move any faster and probably won't stop me from asking you to come more often, but I'll be thankful that I am still part of your life. I hope that you will set time aside for us to visit rather than just fitting me in somewhere because I live for your visits, even if I don't remember them for long once you leave. My mind may betray me; but my spirit knows when you are near, and you make an old woman happy in our times together.

CHAPTER 5

CHRISTMAS IN JUNE— MEET ME WHERE I AM

If I wish you a Merry Christmas in June, feel free to come into my world and let's have some eggnog. You won't be able to talk me out of it or reason it away, so humor me and meet me where I am—and *when* I am. I know a lot of what I am saying these days doesn't make sense, but who cares? We are together, and that's what matters. Let's speak of happy things and people we love, and let's laugh when we can.

This is another example of how I have lost the ability to reason, so correcting me when I am confused won't make me understand. This will only embarrass and confuse me and make me want to withdraw even more. Besides, does it matter that I didn't dance with Pierce Brosnan last night if I think I did? You wouldn't take that piece of happiness away from me, would you? My ramblings now may border on the bizarre, but feel free to see the humor in them.

Jo Huey with the Alzheimer's Caregiver Institute penned "10 Absolutes of Communicating Through Alzheimer's."[1] I share them here in my own words to help you as we travel this road together:

1. Never argue. Instead, agree.

This is going to be a tough one to get used to because you probably won't think you are arguing with me; but if you are correcting me, it will feel to me like you are. You are the one who is going to have to change and swallow the bitter pill of being "wrong" when we disagree because you will be trying to reason with someone who has lost the capacity to do so. This will happen a lot and there is the potential for those exchanges to become heated very quickly, leaving us both frustrated. The easy answer is for you to just agree with me. I will be happy because I am right, and you will be happy about taking the high road on something that doesn't matter and won't change a thing.

2. Never reason. Instead, divert.

I have always been brighter than your average bear but you are learning that I don't shine as brightly and am growing dimmer and dimmer with each passing week. When I say something that is off the wall, remember that reasoning with me is a dead end. Rather, try diverting my attention to something else instead of saying what you know to be true and I cannot know to be true. You can correct me, and may even get me to agree with you; but it won't make a bit

---

[1] *Alzheimer's Disease: Help and Hope*, Jo McDonnell Huey, 2008

of difference a few minutes from now, when I may say the same outrageous thing again.

A common request among those with Alzheimer's disease is to "go home." I first learned about this while dealing with my mom, because she would tell us she wanted to go home while sitting in her home of thirty-seven years. It was distressing for us to think that she didn't feel like she was home, that she did not recognize her surroundings. We would ask her where that home was, but she could never tell us. Was she thinking about her childhood home? Was it one of the homes we lived in along the way? It was frustrating for all of us, and we eventually learned to tell her that we would go after lunch or after she had a nap. By then she would have forgotten about it, at least for the time being.

3. Never shame. Instead, distract.

When you were young and would act unacceptably, I would correct you to teach you not to continue that behavior so you came to understand the principle of cause and effect. Well, that isn't going to work with me. If you shame me for something I do, it will hurt my feelings; but I also won't remember it the next time that doing it seems like a good idea again. Whenever possible, distract me with something that you know I like. Remember that I wasn't above bribery when you were children, and you don't have to be above it now. No judgment!

4. Never lecture. Instead, reassure.

You are going to have many opportunities to lecture me about my language, my incontinence, my forgetfulness, my behavior, and so on. As my motor skills wane and I drop, break and spill things, you may find your frustrations coming to the surface regularly. The adage is true that it is no use crying over spilled milk, and it will go a long way if you remember this and reassure me. When I was a child, I caused many accidents as I learned to master my motor skills. Now those skills are waning, and I am going from being the master back to being the child.

5. Never say "remember when." Instead, reminisce.

It will be difficult for you to remove the words "remember when" from your vocabulary because it is such an easy way to begin a conversation with me. However, it would do us both a favor when you do. My ability to remember has vanished. Instead of saying, "Do you remember when we went to Hawaii?", just start talking about that trip, and either I will join in with my memories or I won't recall it and we can move on. Saying "remember when" will put pressure on me to come up with a memory I can no longer access to and may embarrass me or make me feel inadequate.

6. Never say "I told you." Instead, repeat.

You know that you gave me the answer to my question just three minutes ago, but answering my second (or third or fourth) request is standard for us now, and it is bound to exasperate you. If you keep in mind that I am not obtuse but rather that I sincerely don't remember your answer, it will make it easier for you to respond to me again and again and again with the patience of your first response.

7. Never say "You can't." Instead, do what they can.

When you were little, instead of asking you if you wanted to get dressed, I asked if you wanted to wear the pink outfit or the purple one. This tactic reduced the chance that you would say you didn't want to get dressed at all and allowed you to exercise a small amount of agency. There is much I can no longer do, and it will go a long way if you direct me to what I can do rather than telling me what I can't.

8. Never command. Instead, ask.

We have always been a gracious family, exercising diplomacy at every turn. This is one of the few things that hasn't changed. I may be childlike in many ways now, but asking what you need from me rather than commanding helps me to feel the same love and respect you have always shown me.

9. Never condescend. Instead, encourage.

There will be a lot of people coming in and out of our lives now as the need for doctors, home-care workers, and social workers increases. It will be easy for you to speak to them *about* me rather than *with* me in appointments, and that will make me feel left out and powerless. Include me in the conversations. If I am not able to respond, you can answer questions with what you know and then ask me, 'Is that right Mom?' I am still a real person with real feelings and I respond to respect like everyone else.

10. Never force. Instead, reinforce.

As I lose my abilities, it will be very important for you to take control of situations where I am unable. At those times when I may be confused, scared, or embarrassed, it will make your job easier if you reinforce what I am doing correctly and then work the conversation around to what could be improved. No one likes to be told what to do, so guiding me to a better way should help us all feel good.

It's a new world for me, one I am having a hard time navigating, and one I hope you'll never know firsthand. To keep from losing *your* mind, you will have to accept what we cannot change and learn to live within our new borders. If you constantly correct me, you will only frustrate us all. If you can remember that you are the only one who knows what is really going on, then we can simply enjoy our time together.

It may be that without the constraints of time and lucid thinking, I will have the chance to relive any day I want, over and over again. You can think back to your first day of school; but, in my mind, I am back there living it again. Imagine that! I have so many memories and so much time to live them again with you.

CHAPTER 6

LIAR, LIAR, PANTS ON FIRE

This is a tough passage to write because we have had a lifetime of speaking kindly to each other, and I don't want this to come as a surprise. The progression of my condition pretty much guarantees that I am beginning to experience delusions and that I am more than likely aiming my fear of them at you. If I accuse you of poisoning my food, don't take it as a slap to your culinary skills. If I believe you are lying to me, or if I ask for the items that you "stole," don't take it personally. *This is not me speaking.* I like to think that I could never say something to hurt you; but, the fact is that I probably will, and it already breaks my heart to know it.

Oddly enough, these delusions are common and weirdly similar in those suffering from dementia. I may already be experiencing hallucinations where I will see people or smell something that isn't there. I remember this happening to my mom, who would calmly talk about the man standing in her kitchen. It freaked me out; but if it didn't bother her that he was there, I figured it shouldn't bother me. It will be hard for you to hear some of the things I say or the words I use to say them because they will be foreign coming out of my mouth. You used to tease me because I couldn't say words that I found distasteful, even though they weren't necessarily bad language. You may be hearing those words and even more colorful language in the days ahead. I hope that you will be able to find humor in these situations and not think less of me, knowing that I would faint from embarrassment if I had any idea what I was saying.

It's best not to argue with me when I am accusing you of something because I feel I have been wronged. What I'm experiencing is very real to me even though it seems far-fetched to you. My brain is trying to make sense of the world around me, and it is important that my feelings are respected because you're the only ones who can reason them away. It won't make sense for us to argue about it, and I won't want to be corrected. The best strategy will be to turn my attention to something else and hopefully the man in the kitchen will see himself out.

Proviso: There is a big difference between a harmless hallucination that doesn't bother me and one that does. If I am scared of what I am seeing, stay with me and treat it like it is real for you too. Get professional help immediately because chances are good that my mental confusion has been exacerbated by medicines that are not working properly together or any other number of medical reasons.

If I am convinced something has been stolen, it might be a good idea to replace it for me. There is a good chance that I hid the original one from you and forgot where I put it.

I'm glad our relationship has been so loving because it will help you overlook my delusions now and let you leave behind my hurtful words. I hope this chapter is moot and that I have only happy visions of angels and bunnies and that you always find pleasure in visiting with me; but while I'm hoping for the best, I'm planning for the worst. You need to be aware because this is a real condition that could cause you pain if you are not prepared, and that is the last thing I want.

---·❦· CHAPTER 7 ·❦·---

BEING CARE-FULL

Life is a series of changes that we see progressing in, more or less, the way we have been taught to expect they will, but when dementia enters the picture there will be things you didn't see coming. Some of these changes are insidious, creeping up on you unnoticed until one day you recognize them as being a daily part of our lives and you won't be able to pinpoint when they started. Others will appear quickly and leave you shaking your head wondering what parallel universe you just stepped into.

One of the biggest changes for me is around eating. Breaking bread together has been such a big part of our life that you have undoubtedly noticed my decreased interest in food. I have one friend who was an eat-to-live rather than live-to-eat kind of person, and I considered her a little weird. However, there is much more to this lack of appetite than simply eating less. I can suddenly dislike foods that I once enjoyed, or I may put food into my mouth but forget to swallow. As strange as this sounds, it is very real. Cutlery may become a mystery to me, and I may opt instead to eat with my fingers. (Maybe steer me away from the soup course when this happens.) I may not be able to know when food is too hot and could end up hurting myself, so I need help and a bit of coaching through mealtimes.

If you find that I get agitated more easily, check for these common causes: Am I perhaps uncomfortable from sitting too long in the same position? Has there has been a change in my routine? Have I not been sleeping well? Am I hungry or thirsty, too warm or too cold, or just plain lonely? If I am getting more and more aggressive, make sure my doctor knows about it. I could be having an adverse reaction to my medications. If all of these seem to be in order, then perhaps it is a good time to distract me with a walk outside, if that is feasible, or any other activity or discussion on a subject that you know I like. No matter what works or doesn't, your tone with me will almost always make a difference. A soothing voice, a soft touch, or warm hug can calm me and remind me that I am not in this alone.

Keeping these things in mind will first help you recognize what is going on and then be able to help me when I can't help myself. I wish I had been prepared for these very common changes when they happened to my mom. Since I didn't know to expect them, I was often confused and irritated when they occurred. It was like she became a locked safe and the combination kept changing, leaving us in constant confusion. You are so fortunate to have a heads up about this condition. Hopefully, it will help you both cope with my new world in a way that benefits us all.

Each day that passes finds me a little more dependent on others. I will look to you to love me through this, and together we can make our way. But I do not want you being my caregivers. You both knew you wanted to be hairstylists when you were very young, and you are both gifted with that skill set. There are people out there who want to be caregivers and are very good at it, so let them do their job. They have trained for it and are able to meet my needs without the emotional attachment that you have.

Many of these changes we are talking about will be yours to manage and work with, but there are times when bringing in professional help will be the best way to go. Don't ever feel that you are just passing me off to someone else. There is no judgement around knowing your limits, and it will be the best thing for all of us. There is a price to pay for being my caregivers—everything from you possibly suffering from depression, experiencing poor health due to a compromised immune system, and having it negatively affect your work performance.[2] Don't be martyrs—get help!

Very few people get to become seniors without the help of an assortment of medicines and medical professionals, so it is important that you ensure I receive what I need when I need it. There are home-care services that can come in during the day to make sure I am taking my pills correctly, so please use them. Their coming in and out will be a constant interruption of my days, but I hope that I can see these visits as chances to connect rather than as impositions.

If left to my own devices, I will self-medicate and only take the pills that I want to take for whatever reason makes sense at the time, and we all know that medicine only works when taken consistently.

---

[2] https://www.caregiveraction.org/resources/caregiver-statistics

When I heard the term second childhood, it conjured up images of carefree living filled with a renewed freedom to go where I pleased and do what I wanted when I wanted. Little did I know that it meant going back to wearing diapers and being babysat to keep me from stuffing fifty-dollar bills down the garburator. Our roles have reversed, and you will find me behaving like you did when you were a child. Don't be surprised if I throw a tantrum while insisting you stop treating me like a baby. The irony of you spoon-feeding me dinner while I make this complaint will be completely lost on me, so you will have to appreciate that my mind is telling me one thing while my body is telling me the opposite.

I love you girls, more than anything in this world, which is why I want you to promise me you won't clean my toilets. I want you to spend my money, not your life, on things of this nature. I know you love me and want to help where you can, but life is too short for you to spend your free time picking up after me. I also know that as I get frailer each day, that bathroom is going to look worse and worse, and I don't think there is enough inheritance money to cover the therapy you will need if you take on tasks like this. There are just some things you cannot un-see.

My personal sense of decorum will also suffer, and it may cause some uncomfortable or embarrassing moments for you. I have lived a life of personal modesty; but now as my filters wane, all bets are off. I can stand naked as a jaybird in the living room liked I was raised in a nudist colony. You are going to be astounded at who I let see what God gave me, albeit a lot lower than when He gave it, and you will wonder who this woman is. This is exactly my point because I am no longer the woman you've known. I am not the same mom who sent you back to your room to put on the other half of the miniskirt you were trying to wear to school. Modesty schmodesty! There is no such thing as an inappropriate time for me to verbalize my thoughts anymore, and I only hope that my audible musings don't get you into trouble.

Personal hygiene isn't a high priority for me anymore because I am finding it harder and harder to maneuver in the shower or bath, which offers me less incentive to take care of myself in this way. Granted, I'm not doing a lot, so maybe I don't need it as much. But don't be put off if you find I am only showering once a week. This would have horrified me as well a few years ago, but now it doesn't matter as much as I continue to decline. If we do find ourselves in a situation where you are helping me dress or bathe, we will have to relax in knowing that you will treat me with gentle respect.

While I would be grateful for your care, know that I don't want my hygiene to be your responsibility. If at all possible, please find someone else to help me with this.

A home-care professional in this second childhood will be just as effective, and necessary, as a babysitter was in my first childhood. Having them take care of me will allow you to just care about me.

I fully expect you to keep the promise I made you make when you were a teenager: Always have your tweezers handy to pluck rogue facial hairs! I don't want to turn into the bearded lady and, even though it probably doesn't bother me anymore (especially with my eyesight), help me to maintain my dignity whenever possible. But let's keep that process just between us girls.

I know that this is a lot to manage and can become a burden when trying to fit it into your vibrant and active lives. When I am stomping on your last nerve, take a deep breath and see past this condition and into my humanity. It is not the mother, daughter, sister, and friend that I am who is acting out. It's the disease that has taken hold of me.

My dementia will affect all of us, so it will be important for you to take advantage of support groups to manage the strain. It is good to be around people who understand what you are going through, and you could be a help to someone else in search of a kindred spirit. Caregiving is the hardest job in the world, and you are allowed to take time out when you need it. Never feel guilty about doing this, as self-preservation is so important. The airlines tell you that in an emergency you are to put your mask on first, before assisting others, because they know that if you don't take care of yourself first, you will be no good to anyone else. If not visiting me at times is a good way for you to keep your perspective and make the time we do have together as enjoyable as possible, then take the breaks you need. I may not remember my name, but I do know that I always want what is best for you and I release you to accept that.

I have known people who worked hard with their head down their whole life. One day when retirement came, they finally looked up, and there was very little there for them. They lived their remaining years with so many regrets, reliving their disappointments day after day, often making it hard to be around them. I hope that I have done the work to ensure that my last years are full of unicorns and rainbows because, let's face it, I am making most of it up at this point anyway. Why not err on the side of happiness? Make sure you are doing the same by planning for the future and remembering to live while you're alive. Take a chance or two. Cross something off your bucket list and enjoy your time here on Earth. Have as few coulda, shoulda, wouldas as possible when it is you sitting here. You don't think this will happen to you, but then I never thought it would happen to me either. Do your homework now, while you can, to mitigate this condition as much as possible. Take care of your body, exercise your mind, and stay attuned to God's will for your life. Never forget that eternity awaits all of us. Be ready for it. It won't be Heaven for me if you aren't there.

CHAPTER 8

MITIGATION IS THE KEY

We have come such a long way in understanding dementia and Alzheimer's disease that there is no reason to be ignorant about how to deal with these conditions. More importantly, there is no reason not to mitigate potential cognitive decline. You are probably at an age where you are sure this will never happen to you; but then again, most people think they will be the exception. It's always best to be prepared, so please assume that you are a candidate and do what you can now to stave off these diseases. Even if they come up with a cure, prevention is still the best medicine.

The Alzheimer's Association has published *10 Ways to Love Your Brain*, which describes brain-healthy activities that could help reduce your chances of cognitive decline.[3] I've put my own spin on them for you. Please read each one carefully and see how you can incorporate them into your life. Baby steps can take you a long way.

---

[3] The Alzheimer's Association, 225 N. Michigan Ave. Floor 17 Chicago, IL 60601 https://www.alz.org/help-support/brain_health/10_ways_to_love_your_brain

1. Get enough exercise.

Visit your doctor and find out how much and what kind of exercise is best for you. People with cognitive decline find it harder to perform activities of daily living like bathing, dressing, and eating, and there is evidence to show that exercise may help people to keep doing these basic things for themselves and maintain their independence longer.[4]

2. Challenge your mind through education.

Never stop learning! There is so much out there that we don't know, and you can pick any topic you want to know more about so that you can enjoy the process. Learn something new every day because research shows that doing this will build a brain reserve that could help to balance the damage caused by Alzheimer's or other diseases.[5]

3. Don't smoke.

This one goes without saying. The World Health Organization says that your chance of developing dementia increases by 45% when you smoke and the more you smoke the higher that risk.[6] There is simply no defence for smoking, period.

---

[4] https://www.mcmasteroptimalaging.org/blog/detail/blog/2016/01/14/exercise-and-dementia-what-does-the-latest-research-tell-us

[5] https://www.dementia.org.au/search/node/mental%20exercise

[6] https://www.alz.co.uk/news/smoking-increases-risk-of-dementia

4. Take care of your heart by managing your weight, your blood pressure, and diabetes.

A good thing to keep in mind is that anything good for your heart is good for your brain. We have so much information on how a poor diet affects every part of our lives, and it is never too late to make the changes you need to make a difference in your life. How much better is it to avoid becoming diabetic than to get the diagnosis and live with it forever? Researchers are finding that managing our cardiovascular risks could be a huge step forward in reducing dementia across the board.[7]

5. Protect your head by using your seat belt and wearing a helmet.

Sure, helmet hair isn't cool, but neither is having a halo surgically screwed into your skull because you were too cool to wear one.

6. Eat a healthy, balanced diet.

Hippocrates had it right when he said, "Let food by thy medicine and medicine be thy food." Take care of what you put into your body, making sure it is edifying, strengthening, and good for you. Don't be surprised when your body and mind don't fire on all cylinders when you don't take in premium fuel.

---

[7] https://www.ncbi.nlm.nih.gov/pmc/articles/PMC3547419/

7. Get enough sleep.

"Poor sleep is a risk factor for cognitive decline."[8] Your body is doing repair work the whole time you are sleeping, so make sure you give it the time it needs to recuperate by getting enough zzzzs.

8. Take care of your mental health.

This statement is going to mean something different to everyone, so you need to do some soul searching to discover what it means for you. Talk to your friends, but don't wear them out. There are professionals and support groups who can help you through your struggles. They may be expensive, but it is money well spent when you consider the alternative of living every day carrying your burdens alone. It can be as simple as playing hooky from work and going to a matinee or enjoying a fancy coffee while you shop. It doesn't have to be big, just something that feels good and nurtures your soul.

9. Stay social.

There are studies that show a connection between memory loss and loneliness as well as how having daily contact with friends and family can substantially reduce the risk of dementia.[9] Remember to have some fun in all of this! Let off some steam with your friends and be a hostess yourself. It is another way of exercising your mind and enjoying life in the process.

---

[8] https://www.ncbi.nlm.nih.gov/pmc/articles/PMC4323377/

[9] https://www.aarp.org/health/brain-health/info-11-2008/friends-are-good-for-your-brain.html

10. Challenge your mind through puzzles and games.

Try something new for a while. You didn't know you liked Sudoku until you tried it the first time. There are so many brain-building games and activities available out there that can make this last step so enjoyable!

CHAPTER 9

THE DAY YOU WERE BORN

I know that God made it so that every mother thinks her children are the most beautiful, but you girls truly are. You've grown into kind, loving, responsible women who are as beautiful on the outside as you are on the inside.

Rebecca; that first morning when I woke up to your little face, I understood love in a new way. Words aren't enough to describe how I felt when I held you, and everything else paled in comparison. Taking you home and enjoying you in the days that followed, I remember feeling guilty for having been blessed with so much. You were such an easy baby that I felt I could have written a book on raising children. Little did I know that that had everything to do with your temperament and very little to do with my parenting skills. I enjoyed you so much. I kept your first-grade school picture in a big frame on display because it was taken only two months after we found out it would be just the three of us going forward, and I was terrified of raising you girls by myself. The smile on your face in that picture gave me hope that we were going to be OK. And we were more than OK;

we thrived. When your teacher in high school was surprised to find out that you were in a single-parent home, I took it as a great compliment as your mom and your biggest fan. You have an inner strength that is unique to you. You march to the beat of your own drum—something I was never brave enough to do—and I admire you for it.

Rachel; I thought a second child meant that I would have to divide my love, but you taught me that it multiplied instead. You added so much color to my life, and you challenged me...a lot. I was glad I didn't write that book on parenting because I would have had to eat every word of it, but you were your own person and so full of life. You are so warm and thoughtful and enjoy a flair for life that is all your own. Everyone who meets you walks away feeling special.

> We faced our share of challenges, but we faced them together. When you're frustrated with me now, try to remember who I was when we were going through the trials of life and how we stayed close through them.

I admire you girls for your resilience and for making lemonade from the lemons we were handed. I love you for the way you have treated me with respect even when we disagreed, and for being my friends. I still prefer your company to that of anyone else and I never take for granted how blessed I am to be your mom. I give thanks every day for you and the life we have together. I am so proud of you.

CHAPTER 10

SAYING GOODBYE

I see life going on all around me, but only as a spectator now. I recognized how blessed I was to have all that I did: a loving family, a few good friends and a strong, healthy body. I enjoying so many blessings and I thanked God every day for them.

But this was all the past. My body is betraying me now and, with or without my full mental acuity, I resent it. By now I am more than likely losing most of my family and friends to the ravages of time. Each one is a profound loss, reminding me that my time is coming too. Whoever said, "Everyone wants to go to Heaven, but no one wants to die to get there" summed it up well.

I believe the experience of taking my last breath will be like giving birth to you Rebecca; I was only scared because I had never gone through it before. With you, Rachel, the fear was that it wouldn't be the same as what I believed I knew it to be. My life began anew in different ways the first time I held each of you, and I will begin a new life with that last borrowed breath. I can't remember a time when I was afraid of death. Now with it knocking on my door, I trust that I am embracing it. I am a short time away from seeing the face of God. Think of that: *actually seeing the face of God*. I welcome the relief of setting down this worn-out body and relaxing in the arms of my Creator.

> I was with my mom when she passed from this life, and it was a singular experience of love and loss. If you are not able to be with me when my time comes, don't feel that you let me down. I will leave with a heart full of your love for me, so you will be there with me in spirit if not in body.

I would like a green burial where I can be laid to rest in a shroud and return to the earth naturally. To borrow from a favorite movie, Last Holiday, "I lived my whole life in a box. I don't want to be buried in one." If coming to my resting place gives you peace, then feel free to spend time there but never feel obligated to visit my gravesite. I won't be there, so why should you be? It doesn't matter what other people think; do what is right for you because I know you love me and placing flowers that I can't see serves society's idea of what is proper—not mine.

Don't feel guilty when you feel relief along with sadness when I am gone. I know that I will live on in your hearts because of the love we shared, and a mother couldn't ask for more. If God allows me to watch over you, it really will be Heaven for me. I will happily join your guardian angels, Hank and Crystal, to continue taking care of you. If not, I will wait for you on the other side and look forward to the day we can be together again in a place where all my memories of you will be intact.

AFTERWORD

Like everything else in life, I didn't fully understand or care much about cognitive decline until it affected our family. As she got older, Mom was changing—more than we as a family understood—and I can think back to many times when we could have been more understanding or aware of her. When we got the diagnosis of dementia, we started to learn about it and found the Alzheimer's Society of Alberta to be a great resource for us. Even with our new understanding, actually living with it was constantly demanding and confusing.

It breaks my heart to think of the times when my mom was sitting with our families at the big, bustling dinner table, just picking at the food on her plate and seeming so distant from the festive fellowship around her. We tried to help her engage, but we didn't understand that she was not able to follow the conversation or understand our jokes. We didn't understand the progression of the disease and kept trying to manage it without knowing what she needed. We did the best we could with our limited knowledge and with hearts full of love and respect for her. But sadly, those lessons came at her expense.

Alzheimer's disease and dementia choose their victims seemingly at random, and very few people are ready for it.

With the progress medical science has made in understanding these conditions, not only can we be so much more aware and able to recognize symptoms earlier, but we can lessen their hold on us. Offerings like the Alzheimer's Association's "10 Ways to Love Your Brain" show what we can do every day to keep ourselves in top shape mentally and physically. There are such simple lifestyle changes that can help ward off these maladies as much as possible. When I am working out and struggling for every crunch or lunge, I often wish I had just cut back on the donuts when I had the chance. If I had made better choices when I was younger, I wouldn't be paying the price now. The same can be said for our mental health as we age.

Now is the time to make the choices that will serve us down the road. Let's learn about how to take care of our bodies and minds to give us the best chance of living out our days with crystal clarity, enjoying our family and friends, and being healthy right up to the last breath God lends us.

Appendix I

Stats for Awareness

Dementia now affects more people worldwide than ever before: an estimated 50 million today with another 10 million newly diagnosed each year. Without a medical miracle, the World Health Organization estimates the numbers to rise to 82 million by 2030 and an incredible 152 million by 2050.[10]

- Every day from 2016 to 2034 there will be 1000 people turning 65 years old.[11] The care of many of these seniors falls on their families including feeding, dressing, socializing, dispensing medications and making innumerable appointments for family physicians, eye doctors, and hearing professionals.

---

[10] https://www.who.int/en/news-room/fact-sheets/detail/dementia
[11] https://www.familycaregiversbc.ca/community-resources/statistics-in-family-caregiving/

- In Canada, 25,000 new cases of dementia are diagnosed every year, and it is expected that 937,000 Canadians will be living with it by 2031.[12]
- In 2018, caregivers of people with Alzheimer's or other dementias provided an estimated 18.5 billion hours of informal (that is, unpaid) assistance, a contribution to the nation valued at CDN$233.9 billion.[13]
- The worldwide costs of dementia are estimated at US$818 billion. As a result, if dementia care were a country, it would be the world's 18th-largest economy. If it were a company, it would be the world's largest by annual revenue, exceeding Apple (US$742 billion) and Google (US$368 billion).[14]
- Every sixty-five seconds, someone in the United States develops Alzheimer's. One in three seniors dies with some form of dementia.[15]
- Nearly one-fourth of Alzheimer's and dementia caregivers are "sandwich generation" caregivers, meaning they care both for someone with the disease and a child or grandchild, and more than forty percent of family caregivers report that the emotional stress of their role is high or very high.[16]

---

[12] Prevalence and Monetary Costs of dementia in Canada, Alzheimer Society of Canada (2016)

[13] https://www.alzheimers.net/resources/alzheimers-statistics/

[14] https://alzheimer.mb.ca/about-dementia/disease-stats/

[15] https://www.brightfocus.org/alzheimers/article/alzheimers-disease-facts-figures

[16] https://www.alzheimers.net/resources/alzheimers-statistics

- The average person turning fifty years old right now will spend longer caring for an elderly parent than they did caring for children.[17]
- Ontario and Saskatchewan are the only provinces in Canada that allow eight to twelve weeks of extended leave to care for a family member. Problematically, people with dementia live an average of eight to twelve *years* with symptoms.

---

[17] https://www.familycaregiversbc.ca/community-resources/statistics-in-family-caregiving/

Appendix II

Journaling Prompts

Thank you for taking the time to peek into my experience with dementia. I hope I've shed light on the disease and also provided comfort in knowing that, if this is already part of your life, you are far from alone. The following prompts can help parents preparing for the future to share their legacy with their family and friends. There are also prompts meant for children who want to glean memories from their parents while they can. I pray that peace is your companion throughout this challenging yet meaningful journey.

If you would like to leave your children a pre-dementia love letter or journal, here are some ideas to get you started:

What is the best piece of advice you would like to leave with them?

What are ten words you use to describe your child to others?

What is your favorite vacation memory with them?

What is your greatest hope for them?

What is something you wished you had done together? Take a trip to Paris? Have a dog?

Is there a secret you never shared with them?

Is there a favor you would like to ask of them?

Tell them about the day they were born.

If you could choose your last words to them, what would you say?

What is your biggest regret and why?

What are your end-of-life wishes?

Tell them those things that you think will make you feel comfortable and safe: e.g., holding your hand, sitting with your favorite blanket, listening to classical music, or looking at the picture from your living room.

Tell them the best ways for you to be present with them when you are older and not making sense: e.g., physically touching them, looking at pictures of your life together, or reading to you.

Many dementia symptoms are common and can be expected. Which one would be most unlike you to exhibit, and how can you prepare your child to handle it? Think in terms of language, modesty, socialization.

Is there another way that perhaps wasn't mentioned here to help your child manage the changes you will experience?

What consumed your time and energy when your child was young? Where were the places you needed to be (work, caring for your parents, church, travel)? What were the things you needed to do (taking care of your family, running your own business)? Who were the people you needed to see (family, friends, dependents)? These memories will give your child a fuller appreciation of who you were and what life was like for you. You are able to answer questions they won't know to ask until it may be too late.

What do you wish you had prioritized differently in your life?

How did you feel when you no longer had the commitments that kept you busy and fulfilled?

What was the proudest moment of your life? Why?

If you are a child who would like to capture your parents' memories, here are some ideas to get you started:

What is your earliest memory?

What were your school years like for you?

Who was your best friend growing up?

Tell me about the day I was born.

How did you meet Mom/Dad? Tell me about your courtship.

What was your wedding day like?

What is on your bucket list?

Describe your relationship with your mother, father, and siblings growing up.

What would you do differently if you had the chance to do it again?

Tell me about where you grew up.

What is your best piece of advice for me?

What was your proudest moment and why?

What are your end-of-life wishes?

ACKNOWLEDGMENTS

My gratitude goes to the many who have gone before in trying to make sense of dementia and Alzheimer's disease and left a path for us to follow.

Thank you to Don Loney, my editor, my friend, my cheerleader. Thanks for believing in me even when I didn't. A heartfelt shout out to Faith Farthing of FinalEyes Communications Inc. for making me sound much better than I deserve. Thank you my friend.

Thank you to Jo Huey of Alzheimer's Caregiver Institute whose 10 Absolutes of Communicating Through Alzheimer's is so relevant that celebrities and laypeople alike have claimed authorship.

Thank you to the Alzheimer Society Edmonton for their instruction and support to our family as we waded through these waters.

A heartfelt thank you to the caregivers at Shepherd's Garden in Edmonton, Alberta, for their patience and over-the-top kindness to our family at such an emotional time. You are all angels!

I am so grateful to have my sisters Brenda Welwood, Darlene Newton, and Lauri Holomis who have lived the joy and sadness of dementia along with me. I love you dearly.

Rhonda Hoffman lives in Sherwood Park, Alberta, right around the corner from her daughters.

CPSIA information can be obtained
at www.ICGtesting.com
Printed in the USA
LVHW031130120320
649838LV00002B/73

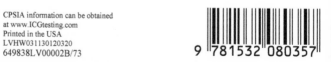